UNRAVELING TRICHOMONIASIS

Navigating Symptoms, Treatment Options, and Preventive Measures

LILIAN NICOLE

CONTENTS

INTRODUCTION

UNDERSTANDING TRICHOMONIASIS

Trichomoniasis is a common sexually transmitted infection (STI) that primarily affects the urogenital tract and is caused by the single-celled protozoan parasite Trichomonas vaginalis. While signs, symptoms, and treatments are important aspects of understanding the infection, delving into its larger context reveals fascinating details about its biology, transmission, and public health impact.

Trichomonas vaginalis, the causative agent of trichomoniasis, is a fascinating microorganism with a distinct structure. It is classified as a flagellated protozoan because it has hair-like structures called flagella that allow it to move. This motility is critical to the parasite's ability to move through the urogenital tract, allowing it to spread during sexual contact.

Trichomoniasis transmission dynamics shed light on its prevalence and risk factors. Unlike some STIs, which can be transmitted in a variety of ways, trichomoniasis is primarily transmitted through sexual contact.

Women are more likely to contract the infection than men, and the risk increases with certain behaviors, such as having multiple sexual partners or engaging in unprotected sex. Understanding these variables is critical for creating effective prevention strategies.

Trichomoniasis has an impact on reproductive and public health outcomes in addition to individual health. In women, the infection has been linked to poor pregnancy outcomes such as preterm birth and low birth weight. Furthermore, trichomoniasis can increase the risk of contracting other STIs, emphasizing its role in the broader landscape of sexual health.

Trichomonas vaginalis' evolutionary aspects add an intriguing layer to its study. For thousands of years, the parasite has coexisted with humans, demonstrating its ability to adapt to its host environment. The study of trichomoniasis' evolutionary history not only sheds light on the dynamics of host-parasite interactions, but it also provides valuable information for developing targeted interventions.

Trichomoniasis prevalence is heavily influenced by social and cultural factors. Stigma surrounding STIs may discourage people from seeking medical attention in a timely manner, resulting in delayed diagnosis and treatment. Addressing these social factors is critical for effective trichomoniasis prevention and control on a larger scale.

Diagnostic tool and technique advancements have played a critical role in our understanding of trichomoniasis. Molecular methods, such as polymerase chain reaction (PCR), have improved parasite detection, allowing for earlier diagnosis and intervention. These advances are critical for increasing the effectiveness of public health initiatives aimed at reducing the trichomoniasis burden.

Trichomoniasis has significant economic implications because the costs associated with diagnosis, treatment, and management of the infection contribute to the overall economic burden of STIs. Investing in preventive measures, such as education and awareness campaigns, has the potential to reduce the economic impact of trichomoniasis by decreasing transmission rates and the need for extensive medical interventions.

Collaboration among healthcare providers, researchers, and policymakers is essential in the global fight against trichomoniasis. Developing comprehensive sexual education programs, promoting regular STI screenings, and ensuring affordable healthcare access are all critical components of a multifaceted global approach to trichomoniasis control.

In conclusion, trichomoniasis is more than just a sexually transmitted infection with distinguishable symptoms and treatments. Exploring its complexities, from fascinating biology to public health implications, provides a comprehensive understanding of the challenges and opportunities in managing this prevalent and persistent parasitic infection. As we continue to decipher the complexities of trichomoniasis, our findings will undoubtedly help to develop more effective prevention and control strategies, ultimately improving sexual health outcomes for individuals and communities worldwide.

CHAPTER ONE

PREVALENCE AND TRANSMISSION

Understanding the prevalence and dynamics of trichomoniasis is essential for developing effective prevention strategies and addressing the broader implications of this often misdiagnosed infection.

Prevalence of Trichomoniasis

Trichomoniasis is one of the most common STIs in the world, with millions of new cases reported every year. However, determining the true prevalence is difficult due to factors such as underreporting, asymptomatic cases, and limited access to healthcare, particularly in resource-constrained settings. While trichomoniasis is widespread worldwide, its prevalence varies by region and population.

The prevalence is higher in women than in men, reflecting both biological and behavioral factors. The parasite thrives in the urogenital environment of women, making them more susceptible to infection. Additionally, asymptomatic cases in both genders contribute to the challenge of accurately estimating the true prevalence of trichomoniasis.

The prevalence of trichomoniasis is influenced by demographic and socioeconomic factors. Individuals with lower socioeconomic status, limited access to healthcare, and a greater number of sexual partners may be more vulnerable. In addition, there are disparities in prevalence across age groups, with younger populations frequently experiencing higher rates of infection.

Transmission Dynamics

Trichomoniasis is primarily transmitted through sexual contact, making it a classic sexually transmitted infection. When an individual comes into direct contact with infected genital secretions, the parasite is transmitted, emphasizing the importance of safe sexual practices in preventing its spread.

Recognizing the roles of asymptomatic carriers and the parasite's persistent nature is a must for understanding the dynamics of trichomoniasis transmission.

Trichomonasis, unlike some STIs, does not require the presence of visible symptoms for transmission. Individuals who are asymptomatic may unknowingly harbor the parasite, acting as reservoirs for infection. This trait contributes to the insidious spread of trichomoniasis within communities and emphasizes the importance of widespread testing to identify and treat both symptomatic and asymptomatic cases.

Men and women have different transmission dynamics. The infection primarily affects the urogenital tract, including the vagina and cervix in women, while the parasite can be found in the urethra and prostate in men. This anatomical variation influences the parasite's ease of transmission during sexual contact.

Beyond individual behaviors, factors influencing transmission include societal and cultural norms. The stigma associated with STIs, including trichomoniasis, may contribute to reluctance to seek medical attention and open communication about sexual health. Addressing these social factors is critical to effective prevention because it creates an environment in which people feel empowered to have candid conversations and seek timely medical attention.

Global Impact and Challenges

Trichomoniasis poses significant global challenges, contributing to the overall STI burden. The impact of the infection on reproductive health, including an association with poor pregnancy outcomes, emphasizes the importance of targeted interventions. Prevalence variations across populations and regions highlight the importance of tailoring prevention and control strategies to specific contexts.

The lack of routine screening, particularly in asymptomatic individuals, makes it difficult to accurately assess the prevalence of trichomoniasis. In a significant proportion of cases, the absence of visible symptoms may result in underdiagnosis and delayed treatment. To overcome these obstacles, a multifaceted approach is required, including increased awareness, routine screening, and the incorporation of sexual education into healthcare initiatives.

Advancement in diagnostic tools, such as nucleic acid amplification tests (NAATs), have improved trichomoniasis detection precision. Access to these diagnostic tools, however, remains a challenge in some regions, hindering efforts to identify and treat cases as soon as possible.

Finally, the prevalence and dynamics of trichomoniasis paint a complex picture shaped by biological, behavioral, and societal factors. Recognizing the global impact of this widespread STI is critical for developing targeted prevention and control strategies. Addressing difficulties in accurate diagnosis, raising awareness, and encouraging open conversations about sexual health are critical steps in reducing the burden of trichomoniasis and promoting overall reproductive well-being.

CHAPTER TWO

TRICHOMONIASIS VS BV

Trichomoniasis and bacterial vaginosis (BV) are two distinct vaginal infections caused by different microorganisms and exhibiting distinct symptoms. While they both affect the vaginal area and are associated with sexual activity, understanding the differences between trichomoniasis and BV is critical for accurate diagnosis and appropriate treatment.

Trichomoniasis:

1. **Causative Agent:** Trichomonasis is caused by the protozoan parasite Trichomonas vaginalis.

2. **Symptoms:** Trichomonasis symptoms include itching, burning, and redness of the genital area, as well as discomfort during urination and sexual intercourse. A distinctive yellow-green, frothy discharge with a strong odor may be present in women.

3. **Transmission:** Trichomoniasis is primarily transmitted through sexual contact. Both men and

women can be infected, with women experiencing symptoms more frequently.

4. **Complications:** Untreated trichomoniasis can result in complications such as preterm birth in pregnant women and an increased susceptibility to other sexually transmitted infections (STIs).

5. **Diagnosis:** Diagnosis frequently involves microscopic examination of a wet mount sample of vaginal or urethral discharge, as well as molecular tests such as polymerase chain reaction (PCR).

Bacterial Vaginosis (BV):

1. **Causative Agents:** BV is caused by an imbalance in the normal vaginal flora, resulting in an overgrowth of harmful bacteria such as Gardnerella vaginalis.

2. **Symptoms:** BV symptoms may include a thin, grayish-white vaginal discharge with a distinct fishy odor. However, up to half of those affected may not exhibit any symptoms.

3. **Transmission:** Although sexual activity can affect the composition of the vaginal flora, BV is not considered a sexually transmitted infection. The precise mechanisms of transmission and factors

contributing to the development of BV are not fully understood.

4. **Complications:** While BV may not cause serious complications, it has been linked to an increased risk of preterm birth, pelvic inflammatory disease (PID), and an increased susceptibility to other STIs.

5. **Diagnosis:** BV is frequently diagnosed using clinical criteria, such as the Amsel criteria (presence of specific vaginal discharge characteristics). Microscopy and pH testing in laboratories may also be used for confirmation.

Distinguishing Factors:

1. **Causative Agents:** Trichomoniasis is caused by a parasitic protozoan, whereas BV is caused by an imbalance in the vaginal bacterial flora.

2. **Symptoms:** Trichomoniasis typically manifests with more noticeable and specific symptoms such as itching, burning, and characteristic discharge. BV, on the other hand, may be asymptomatic in some cases and has milder symptoms.

3. **Transmission:** Trichomoniasis is a sexually transmitted infection with a clear link to sexual

activity. BV is not classified as a STI, and its exact transmission mechanisms are unknown.

4. **Complications:** Trichomoniasis has specific complications, such as an increased risk of preterm birth and susceptibility to other STIs. BV is linked to an increased risk of complications, such as PID and preterm birth.

5. **Diagnosis:** The diagnostic approaches for trichomoniasis and BV differ. Trichomoniasis is frequently confirmed through microscopic examination or molecular tests, whereas BV is diagnosed using clinical criteria and laboratory tests.

In conclusion, while both trichomoniasis and bacterial vaginosis affect the vaginal area and may share some symptoms, they have distinct causative agents, transmission dynamics, and diagnostic criteria. Seeking timely and accurate medical diagnosis is critical for proper management and treatment of these conditions.

TRICHOMONIASIS VS HPV

Trichomoniasis and human papillomavirus (HPV) are distinct infections with distinct causative agents, modes of transmission, and clinical implications. Here's a comparative overview that highlights the key differences between trichomoniasis and HPV:

Trichomoniasis:

1. **Causative Agent:** Trichomoniasis is caused by the protozoan parasite Trichomonas vaginalis.

2. **Transmission:** Trichomoniasis is primarily transmitted through sexual contact. It affects both men and women, but women are more likely to experience symptoms.

3. **Symptoms:** Common symptoms include itching, burning, redness of the genital area, discomfort during urination and sexual intercourse, and, in women, a characteristic yellow-green, frothy discharge with a strong odor.

4. **Complications:** Untreated trichomoniasis can result in complications such as preterm birth in pregnant women and an increased susceptibility to other sexually transmitted infections (STIs).

5. **Diagnosis:** Diagnosis entails microscopic examination of a wet mount sample of vaginal or urethral discharge, as well as molecular tests such as polymerase chain reaction (PCR).

Human Papillomavirus (HPV):

1. **Causative Agents:** HPV is a group of related viruses, and different strains are responsible for different clinical manifestations. Some strains are linked to genital warts (low-risk HPV), while others are linked to cervical and other cancers (high-risk HPV).

2. **Transmission:** HPV is primarily transmitted through direct skin-to-skin contact, which occurs frequently during sexual activity.

3. **Symptoms:** HPV infection can be asymptomatic, and many people recover without showing any symptoms. In some cases, genital warts (low-risk HPV) or Pap smear abnormalities (high-risk HPV) may develop.

4. **Complications:** Long-term high-risk HPV infections can lead to cervical, anal, and other cancers.

Low-risk HPV strains can cause benign growths such as genital warts.

5. **Diagnosis:** Pap smears, HPV DNA testing, or visual inspection for genital warts are all used to diagnose HPV. Routine screening is critical for detecting and managing HPV-related conditions.

Distinguishing Factors:

1. **Causative Agents:** Trichomoniasis is caused by a parasitic protozoan (Trichomonas vaginalis), whereas HPV is caused by a group of DNA viruses with different strains.

2. **Transmission:** Trichomoniasis is primarily a parasitic infection transmitted through sexual contact, whereas HPV is a viral infection transmitted through skin-to-skin contact, including sexual activity.

3. **Symptoms:** Trichomoniasis frequently causes noticeable symptoms, whereas HPV infection can be asymptomatic or manifest as visible warts or abnormal Pap smears.

4. **Complications:** Trichomoniasis complications include preterm birth and increased susceptibility to other STIs. HPV, particularly high-risk strains, can cause cancer.

5. **Diagnosis:** Trichomonasis is diagnosed using microscopy and molecular tests, whereas HPV is diagnosed using Pap smears, HPV DNA testing, or visual inspection.

In conclusion, while both trichomoniasis and HPV are associated with sexual activity, they differ in causative agents, transmission dynamics, symptoms, complications, and diagnostic approaches. Seeking regular healthcare check-ups and screenings is critical for early detection and management of these infections.

TRICHOMONIASIS VS CHLAMYDIA

Both Trichomoniasis and Chlamydia are sexually transmitted infections (STIs), but they are caused by different pathogens and have different symptoms. Here's an outline of each:

Trichomoniasis:

1. **Cause:** Trichomoniasis is caused by Trichomonas vaginalis, a single-celled protozoan parasite.

2. **Symptoms:** Itching, burning, redness, and an unusual discharge are all possible symptoms. However, a significant number of cases, particularly in men, are asymptomatic.

3. **Transmission:** Sexual contact, including vaginal, penile, or vulvar contact, is the primary mode of transmission.

4. **Diagnosis:** Clinical evaluation, laboratory tests (such as wet mount microscopy or nucleic acid amplification tests), and physical examination are all part of the diagnosis process.

5. **Complications:** If trichomoniasis is not treated, it can lead to complications such as an increased risk of other STIs, pregnancy complications, and pelvic inflammatory disease (PID).

Chlamydia

1. **Cause:** Chlamydia is caused by the bacterium Chlamydia trachomatis.

2. **Symptoms:** Like trichomoniasis, Chlamydia can cause no symptoms. Symptoms that do occur include urination pain, abnormal discharge, and pelvic pain. Men can be affected by Urethritis.

3. **Transmission:** Chlamydia is primarily transmitted through sexual contact, which can include vaginal, anal, or oral sex.

4. **Diagnosis:** Diagnosis involves testing swab samples with nucleic acid amplification tests (NAATs).

5. **Complications:** If left untreated, chlamydia can lead to serious complications like pelvic inflammatory disease (PID), infertility, and an increased risk of ectopic pregnancy.

Distinguishing Factors

- A parasite causes trichomoniasis, whereas bacteria cause Chlamydia.

- Trichomoniasis causes itching and redness, whereas Chlamydia causes urination pain and pelvic pain.

- In the early stages, Chlamydia is more likely to be asymptomatic.

- Diagnosis testing methods differ; wet mount microscopy is commonly used to diagnose trichomoniasis, whereas NAATs are used to diagnose chlamydia.

- Both trichomoniasis and chlamydia can cause complications from untreated infections, such as PID and infertility.

Individuals must practice safe sex, get regular screenings, and seek immediate medical attention if they suspect they have trichomoniasis or chlamydia. The importance of early detection and treatment in preventing complications and promoting overall sexual health cannot be emphasized.

CHAPTER THREE

CAUSATIVE AGENT

TRICHOMONAS VAGINALIS

Trichomonas vaginalis is a distinct protagonist in the world of sexually transmitted infections (STIs), orchestrating its presence within the intricate landscapes of the urogenital tract. As a microscopic protozoan parasite, its mode of operation is both stealthy and effective, influencing the lives of millions of people worldwide. This comprehensive overview aims to unravel the many facets of Trichomonas vaginalis, including its biology, transmission dynamics, clinical manifestations, and the broader public health implications.

Unveiling the Parasitic Architect

Trichomonas vaginalis, a single-celled eukaryotic organism from the genus Trichomonas, is at the heart of trichomoniasis. This protozoan navigates its environment with remarkable agility, thanks to its pear-shaped body, undulating membrane, and flagella. Trichomonas vaginalis is only found in the human urogenital tract, where it establishes itself and initiates the chain of events that leads to trichomoniasis.

Transmission Behavior

Trichomoniasis, also known as a "silent epidemic," is primarily transmitted through sexual contact. Intimate bodily fluid exchange facilitates the transmission of Trichomonas vaginalis from an infected individual to an uninfected host. Unlike some STIs that have multiple modes of transmission, trichomoniasis is spread through direct, personal contact.

Trichomonas vaginalis can infect both men and women, but the clinical manifestations and burden of symptoms are often more severe in women. The complex dance of transmission involves the parasite being transferred during sexual activity, where it finds a welcoming environment in the urogenital tract to establish its presence.

Clinical Manifestations

Trichomoniasis manifests in a variety of ways, ranging from obvious symptoms to subtle, almost imperceptible signs. In women, the infection may cause itching, burning sensations, and genital redness. Discomfort during urination and sexual intercourse emerges as a distinguishing feature, emphasizing the parasitic invasion.

The characteristic vaginal discharge of trichomoniasis in women is a yellow-green, frothy secretion with a strong odor. This visual cue frequently prompts people to seek medical attention. Trichomonas vaginalis, on the other hand, does not limit its impact to obvious symptoms; a significant proportion of cases, both in men and women, remain asymptomatic, contributing to the infection's stealthy nature.

In men, symptoms are less severe, and the infection may go undetected for long periods of time. While some men may experience itching or irritation inside the penis, the nuances of these symptoms can lead to delayed diagnosis and possible transmission.

Impacts on Public Health

Beyond the individual experience, trichomoniasis reverberates through public health corridors, with implications that go beyond immediate discomfort. In women, the infection has been linked to poor reproductive outcomes, including an increased risk of preterm birth and low birth weight. These links highlight trichomoniasis's broader impact on maternal and child health.

The economic burden of trichomoniasis is also highlighted when the costs of diagnosis, treatment, and long-term management are considered. Trichomoniasis, as a common STI, adds to the strain on healthcare systems worldwide, necessitating strategic interventions to mitigate its societal impact.

Diagnostic Challenges and Advancements

Despite its prevalence, trichomoniasis faces diagnostic challenges that have historically contributed to underdiagnosis and undertreatment. The reliance on microscopic examination of wet mounts or cultures has limitations, particularly in asymptomatic individuals where the parasite may elude detection.

However, as technology advances, the landscape of trichomoniasis diagnostics evolves. Polymerase chain reaction (PCR), for example, has emerged as a powerful tool with increased sensitivity and specificity. These advancements not only improve diagnostic accuracy, but also play an important role in early detection and intervention, lowering the risk of complications and transmission.

Evolutionary Odyssey

Investigating the evolutionary history of Trichomonas vaginalis reveals an enthralling story of coexistence and adaptation. For millennia, this protozoan parasite has co-evolved with humans, demonstrating its ability to persist and adapt to the ever-changing dynamics of the host-parasite relationship.

Understanding the evolutionary trajectory reveals information about the genetic diversity of Trichomonas vaginalis strains as well as their adaptation to different populations. Exploring the parasite's genetic nuances informs intervention strategies, emphasizing the importance of a nuanced and context-specific approach to trichomoniasis control.

Sexual Health Discourse and Societal Stigma

Trichomoniasis, like many other STIs, is burdened by societal stigma. The unwillingness to discuss sexual health openly contributes to delayed diagnosis and treatment-seeking behavior. Promoting an open dialogue about sexual health is critical for breaking down the barriers that perpetuate misinformation and stigma.

Educational initiatives and stigma-reduction campaigns are critical in changing societal attitudes. Individuals are more likely to seek timely medical care if sexual health conversations are normalized, fostering an environment in which trichomoniasis and other STIs are met with understanding rather than judgment.

Global Prevention and Control Strategies

Tackling the trichomoniasis problem requires a multifaceted approach that goes beyond individual diagnoses and treatments. Comprehensive sexual education programs are critical in raising awareness about safe sexual practices, transmission dynamics, and the value of regular screenings.

Access to affordable healthcare is critical to ensuring that people have the resources to seek medical attention as soon as possible. Furthermore, de-stigmatizing conversations about trichomoniasis and STIs in general contributes to a cultural shift, allowing people to prioritize their sexual health without fear of being judged.

MODE OF INFECTION

Trichomoniasis is primarily transmitted through sexual contact, making it a classic sexually transmitted infection. The causative agent, Trichomonas vaginalis, thrives in the urogenital tract, and transmission occurs when an uninfected person comes into direct contact with infected genital secretions of someone harboring the parasite.

Trichomonas vaginalis is transmitted through the intimate exchange of bodily fluids during sexual activities such as vaginal intercourse, oral sex, and anal sex. Trichomonasis, unlike some other STIs, does not always require the presence of visible symptoms for transmission to occur. Asymptomatic individuals, who may not show any visible signs of infection, can still transmit the parasite to their sexual partners, contributing to the slow spread of trichomoniasis within communities.

CHAPTER FOUR

TRICHOMONIASIS IN MEN

Trichomoniasis, which is commonly thought to be a female-only infection, can also affect men, though the symptoms are more subtle. Trichomoniasis in men is caused by the protozoan parasite Trichomonas vaginalis and has a distinct set of clinical manifestations, transmission dynamics, and reproductive health implications. This in-depth examination delves into the complexities of trichomoniasis in men, shedding light on the signs, symptoms, diagnostic challenges, and potential consequences of this frequently overlooked male reproductive health concern.

Clinical Signs and Symptoms

Trichomoniasis in men often starts with mild or even asymptomatic symptoms, which contributes to underdiagnosis and undertreatment. When symptoms do occur, they usually include the following:

1. **Urethral Discharge**: The presence of a thin, watery, or frothy discharge from the urethra is one of the distinguishing features. This discharge can range in color and consistency from white to yellow-green and can have a noticeable odor.

2. **Irritation and Itching:** Itching or irritation inside the penis may occur in men with trichomoniasis. This discomfort is usually mild, but it can be bothersome, prompting individuals to seek medical attention.

3. **Burning Sensation:** Some men may experience a burning sensation while urinating. This symptom, while not exclusive to trichomoniasis, contributes to the overall discomfort associated with the infection.

4. **Redness and Swelling:** Inflammation of the urethral tissues can cause redness and swelling, adding to the overall discomfort of trichomoniasis patients.

While these are symptoms of trichomoniasis, it is important to note that a significant proportion of men infected with Trichomonas vaginalis may be asymptomatic. Asymptomatic carriers, despite the absence of visible symptoms, can still transmit the parasite to their sexual partners, emphasizing the importance of targeted testing and early intervention.

Transmission Dynamics in Men

Trichomoniasis is primarily transmitted through sexual contact in men, just as it is in women. When an uninfected man has sexual contact with an infected partner, the exchange of genital secretions allows Trichomonas vaginalis to establish itself in the urogenital tract.

In men, the urogenital tract becomes a battleground where the parasite can live, primarily in the urethra and, less commonly, in the prostate. The parasite's presence in these anatomical regions contributes to the localized symptoms that some men experience.

Due to the different physiological environments of the male urogenital tract, men may exhibit fewer symptoms than women, where the infection tends to affect the vagina and cervix more prominently. This subtlety in presentation often results in delayed diagnosis and potential transmission during sexual activity.

Diagnostic Challenges

Diagnosing trichomoniasis in men is difficult, owing to the infection's mild or asymptomatic nature. Many men may not seek medical attention unless they notice symptoms, which contributes to underdiagnosis and the possibility of ongoing transmission.

Traditional diagnostic methods involve microscopic examination of urethral discharge, which may not always produce accurate results, particularly in cases of low parasite density or when individuals are asymptomatic. Cultures and wet mounts are other methods for detecting Trichomonas vaginalis, but they can be insensitive in some cases.

Technological advancements in molecular diagnostic tools, such as polymerase chain reaction (PCR), have increased the accuracy of trichomoniasis detection in both men and women. PCR-based tests have higher sensitivity and specificity, allowing for more precise identification of asymptomatic carriers and prompt intervention.

Complications and Reproductive Health Impact

While trichomoniasis in men is commonly thought to be a minor, self-limiting infection, it is not without consequences. Localized inflammation and irritation in the urogenital tract can cause discomfort and, in rare cases, complications.

Untreated trichomoniasis in men, in particular, has been linked to an increased risk of contracting other sexually transmitted infections (STIs). The inflammatory response elicited by the presence of Trichomonas vaginalis may facilitate the transmission of viruses such as HIV.

Additionally, the potential impact of trichomoniasis on male fertility and reproductive health deserves consideration. Although the evidence is not as extensive as it is in women, there is growing recognition of the potential links between untreated trichomoniasis and negative effects on sperm quality and function. Changes in the urogenital microenvironment may affect sperm motility and viability, potentially affecting male fertility.

TRICHOMONIASIS IN WOMEN

Trichomoniasis represents a common but often underestimated sexually transmitted infection (STI) in women. This comprehensive analysis delves into the complexities of trichomoniasis in women, examining its signs and symptoms, transmission dynamics, diagnostic methods, and potential implications for reproductive health.

Clinical Manifestations

Trichomoniasis in women is characterized by a wide range of clinical manifestations, from obvious symptoms to subtle signs. The following are the most common signs and symptoms:

1. **Vaginal discharge:** The presence of an abnormal vaginal discharge is a defining feature of trichomoniasis. The discharge is usually frothy, yellow-green in color, and has a strong, unpleasant odor. This distinct discharge is frequently a key indicator that leads women to seek medical attention.

2. **Itching and irritation in the vaginal area:** Trichomoniasis can cause vaginal and vulvar itching

and irritation. The pain can range from mild to severe, affecting overall well-being and prompting individuals to seek relief.

3. Genital Swelling and Redness: The presence of Trichomonas vaginalis can cause inflammation of the genital tissues, resulting in redness and swelling. This adds to the discomfort felt by those who are affected.

4. Discomfort during Urination and Sexual Interaction: Trichomoniasis can cause pain and discomfort during urination and sexual contact. Irritation and inflammation in the urogenital tract contribute to these symptoms, lowering people's quality of life.

It's important to note that not all women with trichomoniasis have visible symptoms. Asymptomatic cases are common, complicating the diagnosis and transmission dynamics of the infection. While asymptomatic carriers may not show obvious symptoms, they can still transmit the parasite to sexual partners, emphasizing the importance of targeted testing and education.

Transmission Dynamics in Women

Trichomonasis is primarily transmitted to women through sexual contact, including vaginal intercourse. When an uninfected woman has sexual contact with an infected partner, the exchange of genital secretions allows Trichomonas vaginalis to settle in the urogenital tract.

Trichomonas vaginalis primarily affects the female lower genital tract, including the vagina and cervix. The parasitic invasion can cause inflammation, disrupting the normal microenvironment and causing the typical trichomoniasis symptoms.

Transmission can occur even when the infected person is asymptomatic, emphasizing the importance of routine testing, especially in populations with higher risk factors or individuals who have multiple sexual partners.

Diagnostic Methods

Trichomonasis in women is diagnosed through a combination of clinical and laboratory testing. The following diagnostic techniques are commonly used:

1. Microscopic Examination: A traditional method for identifying Trichomonas vaginalis is microscopic examination of a wet mount preparation of vaginal or cervical discharge. Under a microscope, the parasite's characteristic motility can be seen. This method, however, may be insensitive, especially in cases of low parasite density or when women are asymptomatic.

2. Culture: Culturing urogenital tract samples allows for the growth and identification of Trichomonas vaginalis. Culture methods, while more sensitive than microscopic examination, can take several days to produce results.

3. Nucleic Acid Amplification Tests (NAATs): Molecular diagnostic techniques such as polymerase chain reaction (PCR) have transformed the testing of trichomoniasis. Because NAATs have high sensitivity and specificity, they can detect Trichomonas vaginalis DNA even in cases of low parasite density or asymptomatic carriage. PCR-based tests have evolved into valuable diagnostic tools for accurate and timely diagnosis.

Routine trichomoniasis screening is especially important for early detection and intervention, preventing complications and lowering the risk of transmission.

Impact on Reproductive Health and Complications

While trichomoniasis is generally thought to be a curable infection, untreated cases in women can lead to complications and have an impact on reproductive health. Among the most important considerations are:

1. Increased Probability of Other STIs: Untreated trichomoniasis may increase the risk of contracting other sexually transmitted infections (STIs), such as HIV. Inflammation and changes in the urogenital microenvironment can make the environment more conducive to virus transmission.

2. Undesirable Pregnancy Outcomes: Trichomoniasis during pregnancy has been linked to a higher risk of preterm birth and low birth weight. For mitigating these risks and promoting optimal maternal and fetal health, early detection and treatment are critical.

3. PID (Pelvic Inflammatory Disease): Although trichomoniasis is less common than other STIs, it can contribute to the development of pelvic inflammatory disease (PID). PID causes inflammation of the reproductive organs and can lead to long-term complications such as infertility.

CHAPTER FIVE

ASYMPTOMATIC CASES

Trichomoniasis is commonly associated with symptoms such as itching, burning, and discharge. However, a significant number of trichomoniasis patients are asymptomatic, complicating detection and potentially leading to the infection's inadvertent spread.

Asymptomatic cases of trichomoniasis pose a unique public health challenge. While the absence of visible symptoms may provide infected individuals with a false sense of security, it does not diminish the potential health risks associated with the condition. Understanding the characteristics, prevalence, and consequences of asymptomatic trichomoniasis is critical for effective prevention and management.

The absence of overt clinical signs is one of the defining features of asymptomatic trichomoniasis. In contrast to symptomatic infections, in which individuals may experience vaginal itching, discomfort during urination, or abnormal discharge, those with asymptomatic infections may be unaware of their condition. This lack of awareness may contribute to the unintentional transmission of the parasite to sexual partners.

According to prevalence studies, a sizable proportion of trichomoniasis cases are asymptomatic. The actual figures vary by population, but research indicates that up to half of infected people may not show any symptoms. This high prevalence of asymptomatic cases emphasizes the importance of routine screening, particularly in high-risk groups, to identify and treat infections as soon as possible.

The reasons for the asymptomatic nature of trichomoniasis in some people are unknown. Some believe that host immune responses play a role in determining whether an infection causes symptoms. Variations in the virulence of different Trichomonas strains may also contribute to differences in clinical presentation.

The consequences of untreated asymptomatic trichomoniasis are far-reaching. While the absence of symptoms may appear to be benign, the infection can have serious consequences for reproductive and overall health. Untreated trichomoniasis in women has been associated with an increased risk of preterm birth, low birth weight, and susceptibility to other STIs, including HIV.

In men, the infection has been linked to urethritis and may contribute to HIV transmission.

The challenge in treating asymptomatic trichomoniasis stems from its invisibility. Routine screening becomes critical, especially in populations with a higher prevalence of STIs. Testing methods such as nucleic acid amplification tests (NAATs) and polymerase chain reaction (PCR) have proven effective in detecting Trichomonas infections even in the absence of symptoms.

Educational campaigns are important in raising awareness about the asymptomatic nature of trichomoniasis. Regular STI screenings, regardless of symptoms, can help identify and treat infections early, preventing complications and interrupting the chain of transmission.

Furthermore, promoting safe sexual practices remains a cornerstone of trichomoniasis prevention. Consistent and proper condom use can significantly reduce the risk of transmission. Open communication about sexual health between partners fosters an environment in which testing and treatment are normalized, reducing the stigma associated with STIs.

Healthcare providers play a critical role in treating asymptomatic trichomoniasis. Routine STI screenings during routine check-ups, particularly for people who have multiple sexual partners or live in high-prevalence areas, can help identify asymptomatic cases. Counseling on safe sex practices and the importance of regular screenings further empowers individuals to take charge of their sexual health.

Finally, asymptomatic cases of trichomoniasis pose a complex challenge in the realm of sexual health. The lack of obvious symptoms makes detection more difficult and may contribute to the unintentional spread of the infection. Addressing this issue requires a multifaceted approach that includes routine screenings, educational campaigns, and open communication about sexual health. We can work to reduce the impact of asymptomatic trichomoniasis on reproductive and overall health by better understanding and managing it.

THE IMPORTANCE OF TESTING FOR ACCURATE DIAGNOSIS

Accurate testing for trichomoniasis is critical, especially in asymptomatic cases, as it plays an important role in both individual healthcare and public health strategies. Several key reasons highlight the importance of testing for accurate diagnosis in asymptomatic trichomoniasis cases:

1. Identification of Asymptomatic Infections: Asymptomatic individuals may unknowingly carry and transmit the Trichomonas parasite. Testing allows for the detection of these silent infections, preventing the disease's inadvertent spread.

2. Preventing Complications: Asymptomatic trichomoniasis can lead to severe complications, particularly in women. Early detection through testing allows for early intervention and treatment, lowering the risk of adverse outcomes such as preterm birth, low birth weight, and increased susceptibility to other sexually transmitted infections, including HIV.

3. Interrupting Transmission: Identifying and treating asymptomatic cases is critical in breaking the chain of transmission. Individuals may be unaware of their infection status if accurate testing is not performed, perpetuating the spread of trichomoniasis within sexual networks.

4. Targeted Treatment: Accurate diagnosis ensures that individuals receive appropriate and targeted treatment. Tailoring treatment regimens based on confirmed test results improves therapeutic outcomes and lowers the risk of drug resistance.

5. Public Health Surveillance: Testing provides critical data for public health surveillance. Understanding the prevalence of asymptomatic trichomoniasis in specific populations allows health officials to implement targeted interventions, allocate resources effectively, and design preventive strategies.

6. Sexual Health Education: Testing can be used to educate people about sexual health. When individuals are informed of their infection status, it provides an opportunity for healthcare providers to discuss safe sex practices, the importance of regular screenings, and overall sexual health awareness.

7. Reducing Stigma: Accurate testing helps to de-stigmatize trichomoniasis by emphasizing that it is a common and treatable infection. This, in turn, encourages people to seek testing without fear of being judged, fostering a more open dialogue about sexual health.

8. Partner Notification and Treatment: Positive test results allow healthcare providers to initiate partner notification and treatment. Notifying sexual partners of potential exposure is essential for preventing reinfection and further transmission within sexual networks.

9. Monitoring Treatment Efficacy: Follow-up testing allows healthcare providers to assess the effectiveness of treatment. Individuals are monitored after treatment to ensure that the infection has been successfully cleared, reducing the likelihood of recurrence.

10. Global STI Control Efforts: Accurate diagnosis contributes to global efforts to control and reduce the burden of sexually transmitted infections. Healthcare systems can make significant strides in overall STI prevention and management by addressing asymptomatic trichomoniasis with effective testing.

In conclusion, accurate testing for trichomoniasis in asymptomatic cases is a cornerstone of comprehensive sexual health care. It enables early detection, targeted treatment, and the implementation of preventive measures, ultimately reducing the impact of trichomoniasis on both individual and public health.

CHAPTER SIX

DIAGNOSIS OF TRICHOMONIASIS

Trichomoniasis is diagnosed through a combination of clinical examination, laboratory testing, and, in some cases, imaging.

The following are some of the primary methods for diagnosing trichomoniasis:

1. Wet Mount Microscopy: Wet mount microscopy is a quick and easy way to diagnose trichomoniasis. A vaginal or urethral discharge sample is collected, mixed with saline, and examined under a microscope. Infection is indicated by the presence of motile, pear-shaped trichomonads with flagella. While this technique produces quick results, it may be less sensitive than molecular methods.

2. Partner Screening: Given trichomoniasis is transmitted sexually, partner screening is critical for effective management. If a person is diagnosed with trichomoniasis, their sexual partner(s) should be tested and treated at the same time to avoid reinfection and further transmission.

3. Imaging Studies: Imaging studies may be used in some cases, particularly when complications or coexisting conditions are suspected. Pelvic ultrasound is a useful tool for assessing pelvic organs and detecting any abnormalities caused by trichomoniasis.

4. Point-of-Care Tests: Rapid point-of-care tests are intended for quick and easy diagnosis in clinical settings. Nucleic acid hybridization and immunochromatographic assays provide immediate results. While they are convenient, their sensitivity varies and they are not as accurate as laboratory-based tests.

5. Antigen Detection Tests: Antigen detection tests identify specific Trichomonas vaginalis proteins. These tests are usually quick and can be done with vaginal swabs. Although they provide faster results, their sensitivity may be lower than that of nucleic acid amplification tests (NAATs) or culture.

6. NAATs (Nucleic Acid Amplification Tests): NAATs, which include polymerase chain reaction (PCR) and transcription-mediated amplification (TMA), are highly sensitive and specific molecular methods for detecting Trichomonas vaginalis genetic material. These tests can be run on a variety of sample types, yielding reliable and accurate results. NAATs have become the gold standard in trichomoniasis diagnosis, particularly in detecting asymptomatic cases.

7. Culture: To culture Trichomonas vaginalis, a sample is placed in a specialized culture medium. While this method is extremely specific, it is less sensitive than other diagnostic techniques and can take several days to produce results. Culture is frequently reserved for situations in which NAATs are unavailable.

8. Microscopic Examination: In addition to wet mount microscopy, microscopic examination includes more specialized techniques such as fluorescent antibody staining. These techniques improve trichomonad visibility and aid in accurate diagnosis.

9. Physical Examination: A physical examination, including a pelvic exam for women, can reveal visible signs of infection like redness, swelling, or discharge. While not definitive, it does provide useful clinical information.

10. Clinical Assessment: The diagnostic process is guided by a comprehensive clinical assessment that takes into account the individual's medical history and reported symptoms. Based on the patient's specific circumstances, it assists healthcare providers in determining the most appropriate tests and procedures.

Finally, trichomoniasis is diagnosed using a combination of laboratory tests and clinical assessments. The method chosen is determined by factors such as availability, cost, and the specific clinical scenario. Combining multiple diagnostic approaches improves accuracy, ensuring timely and effective trichomoniasis infection management. Regular screenings and partner involvement are critical in preventing the infection's spread and potential complications.

CHAPTER SEVEN

MEDICAL TREATMENTS FOR TRICHOMONIASIS

Trichomoniasis requires prompt and effective medical treatment. The most common trichomoniasis medications are metronidazole and tinidazole.

In this chapter, we will look at these prescription medications, their mechanisms of action, and provide detailed dosage and administration instructions.

Prescription Medications

1. Metronidazole:

Mechanism of Action: Metronidazole is a nitroimidazole antibiotic that works by disrupting the DNA of the infecting organism. It enters the bacterial or protozoan cell and is reduced by intracellular electron transport proteins to produce cytotoxic radicals. These radicals cause DNA strand breaks, resulting in cell death and pathogen elimination.

Dosage and Administration: The standard oral dosage for metronidazole in the treatment of trichomoniasis is a single 2-gram dose or divided doses totaling 2 grams taken as a single dose or over the course of a day. Alternatively, a lower dose of 500 mg twice daily for seven days may be prescribed. Metronidazole can also be administered intravaginally to those who cannot tolerate oral medication.

Special Considerations:

Pregnant women are frequently prescribed a longer course of metronidazole treatment. A seven-day regimen of 500 mg twice daily is commonly recommended. However, pregnant women should consult with their healthcare provider to determine the best treatment plan for them, taking into account potential risks and benefits.

 - Alcohol should be avoided during metronidazole treatment and for at least 48 hours after finishing the course. When metronidazole is combined with alcohol, a disulfiram-like reaction occurs, causing nausea, vomiting, and headache.

2. Tinidazole:

Mechanism of Action: Tinidazole, like metronidazole, is a nitroimidazole derivative with a mechanism of action involving the generation of cytotoxic radicals. These radicals cause DNA damage in susceptible organisms, resulting in their extinction.

Dosage and Administration: Tinidazole is an alternative medication for trichomoniasis that is commonly prescribed as a single 2-gram oral dose. The simplicity in dosing makes it a convenient option for patients. Tinidazole, like metronidazole, can be administered intravaginally to those who are unable to take oral medication.

Special Considerations: Tinidazole may be more tolerable in some people than metronidazole, and it has a longer half-life, allowing for a shorter treatment duration with a single high dose.

- As with metronidazole, alcohol should be avoided during tinidazole treatment and for at least 72 hours after finishing the course. When tinidazole is combined with alcohol, it can cause similar disulfiram-like reactions.

Guidelines for Dosage and Administration

1. General Dosage Guidelines:

When determining the appropriate dosage for trichomoniasis treatment, healthcare providers consider a number of factors, including the severity of the infection, patient characteristics, and medical history.

- Single-dose regimens, such as a one-time 2-gram dose of metronidazole or tinidazole, are frequently preferred due to their simplicity and patient compliance.

- For those who are unable to tolerate a single high dose, a longer course of treatment with lower daily doses, such as 500 mg twice daily for seven days, may be recommended.

2. Special Populations:

Pregnant Women:

Pregnant women with trichomoniasis may require special consideration in determining the best treatment plan. To minimize potential risks, extended courses of medication, such as seven days of metronidazole at a lower dose, are commonly prescribed.

Children:

Trichomoniasis is uncommon in prepubertal children, and treatment recommendations may differ. Pediatric dosages are determined by weight and are typically lower than those used in adults.

Individuals with compromised immune systems may require individualized treatment plans. In this population, healthcare providers may opt for longer courses or more closely monitor treatment response.

3. Administration Considerations:

Oral Administration: Oral administration is the standard route for both metronidazole and tinidazole. Medication is usually taken with food to reduce gastrointestinal side effects.

-Intravaginal Administration: Metronidazole and tinidazole can be administered intravaginally when oral medication is not an option. Vaginal formulations are available, and healthcare providers may provide specific administration instructions.

-Alcohol Avoidance: Patients are strongly advised to avoid alcohol consumption during and after metronidazole or tinidazole treatment. Combining these medications with alcohol can cause a disulfiram-like reaction, resulting in unpleasant symptoms.

4. Follow-up and Retesting: It is critical for individuals to follow up with their healthcare provider for retesting after completing the prescribed course of medication to ensure the infection is successfully eradicated. This step is especially important for preventing reinfection and monitoring treatment efficacy.

- Sexual partners should also be informed and encouraged to seek testing and treatment as needed to prevent further transmission.

Finally, metronidazole and tinidazole are the primary prescription medications used in the medical treatment of trichomoniasis. The choice of these medications, as well as the specific dosage and administration plan, is determined by a number of factors, including the patient's medical history, preferences, and the severity of the infection.

Healthcare providers play a critical role in tailoring treatment plans to individual needs, ensuring optimal efficacy while minimizing potential side effects. Regular follow-up and partner involvement are essential components of comprehensive trichomoniasis management. Individuals should, as with any medical treatment, follow prescribed regimens, avoid alcohol as directed, and actively participate in post-treatment monitoring to promote overall health and well-being.

CHAPTER EIGHT

PARTNER TREATMENT IN TRICHOMONIASIS

Trichomoniasis is a sexually transmitted infection that affects not only individuals but also their sexual partners. When one partner is diagnosed with trichomoniasis, treating both partners is a key aspect of comprehensive infection management.

The significance of partner treatment can be understood through the following key points:

1. Preventing Reinfection: Considering the fact that trichomoniasis is highly contagious, there is a risk of reinfection if only one partner receives treatment. The untreated partner may serve as a parasite reservoir, resulting in a cycle of transmission between partners. Treating both individuals at the same time breaks the cycle, lowering the likelihood of recurrent infections.

**2. Interfering with Transmission within Sexual
Networks:** Sexual partners have an intimate
connection, and untreated infections can be easily
transmitted between them. By treating both partners,
healthcare providers help to break the transmission
chain not only between the couple but also across
larger sexual networks. This is especially important
for preventing the spread of trichomoniasis in
communities.

3. Treating Asymptomatic Infections:
Trichomoniasis can be asymptomatic in some people,
which means they don't have any symptoms. If only
one partner is symptomatic and seeks treatment, the
other may be unaware of their infection status. By
treating both partners, asymptomatic infections are
identified and treated, promoting the overall health of
the individuals involved.

4. Comprehensive STI Management:
Trichomoniasis patients may be at risk of other
sexually transmitted infections (STIs). Healthcare
providers take a proactive approach to
comprehensive STI management by treating both
partners. Screening for additional infections,
providing appropriate treatment, and promoting
overall sexual health are all part of this.

5. Building Trust and Mutual Responsibility:
Within relationships, partner treatment fosters an environment of trust and mutual responsibility. Addressing STIs as a group promotes open communication about sexual health, stigma reduction, and a shared commitment to maintaining a healthy sexual environment. This collaborative approach is critical for both partners' well-being and the longevity of their relationship.

Communication and Support

When it comes to trichomoniasis partner treatment, effective communication and support are critical. This includes not only communicating the importance of concurrent treatment, but also providing a supportive and nonjudgmental environment for individuals to discuss their sexual health.

Here are some key points to consider:

1. Encourage Open Dialogue: It is important to encourage open dialogue between partners. Healthcare providers should emphasize the importance of open communication about sexual health issues, including the possibility of trichomoniasis exposure and diagnosis. Providing a safe space for people to express their concerns promotes trust and a collaborative approach to treatment.

2. **Education on Trichomoniasis:** It is essential to provide clear and accurate information about trichomoniasis. Many people are unfamiliar with the infection, its symptoms, and the significance of partner treatment. Educating both partners about trichomoniasis dispels myths, reduces anxiety, and encourages a proactive approach to dealing with the infection.

3. **Empathy and Non-Judgemental Support:** Healthcare providers play a critical role in providing compassionate, non-judgmental support. Recognizing the emotional aspects of a trichomoniasis diagnosis, as well as the potential impact on relationships, can help individuals feel understood and supported. This strategy is especially important for reducing stigma and promoting overall well-being.

4. **Practical Guidance:** Providing practical guidance on the treatment process, such as medication

administration, potential side effects, and post-treatment precautions, ensures that both partners are well-informed and can participate actively in their care. Addressing any concerns or questions helps individuals feel empowered in their health management.

5. Confidentiality: It is essential to emphasize the confidentiality of healthcare information. Individuals may be hesitant to discuss STIs due to privacy concerns. Assuring confidentiality and explaining the legal and ethical standards that protect patient information promotes trust and open communication.

6. Follow-up Care: It is extremely important to develop a follow-up care plan. This includes scheduling post-treatment check-ups for both partners to ensure the infection is successfully eradicated. Follow-up care allows you to address any remaining concerns, retest if necessary, and reinforce future preventive measures.

7. Community Resources: Connecting people with community resources such as sexual health clinics, support groups, or educational materials can improve the overall support system. These resources can provide additional information, counseling services, and opportunities for people to connect with others who have gone through similar experiences.

Finally, partner treatment for trichomoniasis is an essential component of comprehensive STI management. Partner treatment promotes open communication, trust, and mutual responsibility within relationships, in addition to its clinical significance in preventing reinfection and interrupting transmission. Healthcare providers play an important role in facilitating this process by providing clear information, compassionate support, and practical advice.

 Individuals and their partners can navigate trichomoniasis treatment with resilience and contribute to the larger goal of promoting overall well-being by fostering a collaborative approach to sexual health.

CHAPTER NINE

PREVENTION STRATEGIES

While effective treatment is available, prevention strategies play an important role in reducing the prevalence of trichomoniasis and minimizing its impact on individuals and communities.

Here, we take a look at comprehensive prevention strategies that include education, safe sexual practices, and regular screenings.

1. Education and Awareness:

A. Understanding transmission: Knowledge is a powerful tool for preventing trichomoniasis. Individuals and communities require accurate information about how the infection spreads. Understanding that trichomoniasis is primarily transmitted through sexual contact, including vaginal, penile, or vulvar contact, allows people to make more informed decisions about their sexual health.

B. Recognizing Symptoms: It is essential to educate people about trichomoniasis symptoms. While some people experience itching, burning, or discharge, a large number of cases are asymptomatic. The potential absence of symptoms underscores the importance of routine screenings, especially for those at higher risk, such as people who have multiple sexual partners.

C. Partner Treatment: Emphasizing the importance of partner treatment is critical in prevention efforts. When one partner is diagnosed with trichomoniasis, both individuals should seek treatment at the same time to prevent reinfection and break the transmission cycle. Education about partner treatment promotes open communication about sexual health in relationships.

2. Safe Sexual Practices:

A. Condom Use: Using condoms correctly and consistently is an effective preventive measure against trichomoniasis. Condoms act as a barrier, lowering the risk of transmission during sexual activity. Encouragement of condom use, particularly in new or casual sexual relationships, contributes to a safer sexual environment.

B. Monogamy and Mutual Testing: Engaging in monogamous relationships and mutually testing for STIs before sexual activity can be a proactive approach to prevention. Knowing one's own and a partner's STI status allows people to make more informed decisions about their sexual health and reduces the risk of introducing infections into relationships.

C. Communication and Consent: Open communication about sexual health, desires, and boundaries is essential. Establishing clear consent and negotiating safe sexual practices contribute to a respectful and consensual sexual environment. Healthy communication lowers the risk of engaging in behaviors that may result in the transmission of STIs.

3. Routine Screenings:

A. Regular STI Testing: Routine screenings for STIs, including trichomoniasis, are critical for early detection and treatment. Individuals who have multiple sexual partners or engage in high-risk behaviors should prioritize regular testing. Screening allows for the identification of asymptomatic cases, reducing the risk of complications and preventing further transmission.

B. Comprehensive Sexual Health Check-ups: Incorporating comprehensive sexual health check-ups into regular healthcare routines allows individuals to discuss their sexual health with healthcare providers. These check-ups may include discussions about STI prevention, testing, and overall sexual well-being.

4. Community Outreach and Support:

A. Educational Campaigns: Community outreach programs and educational campaigns play a critical role in prevention. Disseminating information through various channels, such as schools, healthcare facilities, and online platforms, raises awareness about trichomoniasis, its transmission, and available prevention strategies.

B. Accessible Healthcare Services: Access to affordable and accessible healthcare services is critical. Individuals should be able to seek testing and treatment without difficulty. Community health clinics, sexual health centers, and other healthcare facilities play an important role in providing services and information to diverse populations.

C. Support Groups and Counseling:

- Support groups and counseling services can help with the emotional and psychological aspects of dealing with STIs. Individuals diagnosed with trichomoniasis may face stigma or anxiety, and having access to supportive environments can contribute to overall well-being and resilience.

5. Personal Hygiene Practices:

A. Hygienic Practices: While not a direct preventive measure, maintaining personal hygiene can help with overall sexual health. Bathing on a regular basis, changing underwear on a regular basis, and avoiding douching may all contribute to a healthy genital environment.

Finally, addressing trichomoniasis requires a multifaceted approach to prevention. Education, safe sexual practices, routine screenings, community outreach, and easily accessible healthcare services all help to reduce the incidence of trichomoniasis and promote overall sexual health. Communities can work to create a safer and healthier environment for all by empowering individuals with knowledge, fostering open communication, and providing support.

CHAPTER TEN

COMPLICATIONS AND RISKS OF TRICHOMONIASIS

Untreated trichomoniasis can cause various kinds of complications, affecting both reproductive and overall health. In this analysis, we look into the long-term health implications of untreated trichomoniasis.

A. Potential Consequences of Untreated Trichomoniasis:

1. Increased Risk of Other STIs: Untreated trichomoniasis may increase the risk of contracting other sexually transmitted infections (STIs). The inflammation caused by Trichomonas vaginalis can create an environment conducive to the transmission of additional pathogens during sexual activity. Individuals with untreated trichomoniasis may be more susceptible to infections such as HIV and herpes.

2. Pregnancy Complications: Trichomoniasis poses special risks to pregnant women. Untreated infections have been associated to an increased risk of preterm birth, low birth weight, and premature membrane rupture. The inflammatory response caused by the infection may contribute to poor pregnancy outcomes, emphasizing the importance of early detection and treatment during pregnancy.

3. Transmission to Sexual Partners: Individuals with untreated trichomoniasis may unknowingly transmit the infection to their sexual partners. Because the infection often presents asymptomatically, the risk of unintentionally spreading Trichomonas vaginalis is higher. It is critical to treat both partners simultaneously in order to break the transmission cycle and prevent reinfection.

4. Pelvic Inflammatory Disease (PID): Trichomoniasis can spread from the lower to upper genital tract, potentially leading to pelvic inflammatory disease (PID) in women. PID is a serious complication that can cause inflammation and scarring of the reproductive organs. Chronic pelvic pain, fertility issues, and an increased risk of ectopic pregnancy are some of the consequences of PID.

5. Urethritis in Men: Untreated trichomoniasis in men can result in urethritis, or inflammation of the urethra. Urethritis can cause pain when urinating, discharge from the penis, and contribute to the spread of the infection. Preventing complications in both men and their sexual partners requires prompt treatment.

6. Vaginal Discomfort and Irritation: In women, persistent trichomoniasis can cause chronic vaginal discomfort and irritation. The parasite's presence may cause recurring symptoms such as itching, burning, and abnormal discharge. It is critical to address the infection as soon as possible in order to alleviate these symptoms and avoid long-term discomfort.

B. Long-Term Health Implications:

1. Recurrent Infections: People with untreated trichomoniasis may experience recurrent infections. The persistent presence of Trichomonas vaginalis can result in a cycle of reinfection, especially if both partners are not treated at the same time. Recurrent infections can contribute to ongoing health problems and complications.

2. Chronic Inflammation and Immune Response:
Chronic trichomoniasis may contribute to long-term inflammation of the genital and reproductive organs. Prolonged inflammation can continuously activate the immune system, resulting in immune response issues. Chronic inflammation has been linked to a variety of health problems, including autoimmune disorders and an increased risk of other infections.

3. Impact on Sexual Health and Relationships:
Trichomonasis can have a long-term impact on sexual health and intimate relationships. Persistent symptoms, discomfort, and the possibility of recurrent infections can lead to sexual dissatisfaction and strain on relationships. Open communication about sexual health, regular screenings, and prompt treatment are critical to overall well-being.

4. Fertility Issues: Untreated trichomoniasis and its complications, such as PID, can contribute to fertility problems in women. Scarring and damage to the reproductive organs may impair fertility, making it more difficult for people to conceive. Early detection and treatment are critical in mitigating these risks.

5. Impact on Reproductive Organs: Long-term trichomoniasis can cause reproductive organ damage in both men and women. In women, this can manifest as scarring of the fallopian tubes, increasing the risk of ectopic pregnancy. In men, inflammation of the reproductive structures may contribute to infertility.

Psychological Impact.

 Living with untreated trichomoniasis can have psychological consequences. The stigma associated with STIs, concerns about transmitting the infection to partners, and the emotional toll of ongoing symptoms can all lead to stress, anxiety, or depression. Integrating mental health support into comprehensive STI care is critical for overall well-being.

Conclusion

The complications and risks of untreated trichomoniasis extend beyond the immediate symptoms, affecting reproductive and overall health. Recognizing the potential consequences, such as increased susceptibility to other STIs, pregnancy complications, and the risk of transmitting the infection to sexual partners, emphasizes the importance of early detection and comprehensive treatment. Long-term health consequences, such as fertility issues and the psychological impact of living with an untreated STI, highlight the need for a comprehensive approach to sexual health. Timely screenings, open communication, and access to healthcare services are critical in mitigating the risks of trichomoniasis and promoting the well-being of individuals and communities.

CHAPTER ELEVEN

20 FAQs AND ANSWERS ABOUT TRICHOMONIASIS

This chapter provides in-depth information about this sexually transmitted infection. Common questions are addressed, from symptoms to prevention, ensuring accurate information for informed health decisions.

Here are some frequently asked Trichomoniasis questions:

1. What exactly is trichomoniasis?

Trichomoniasis is an infection transmitted through sexual contact caused by the protozoan parasite Trichomonas vaginalis.

2. How is trichomoniasis spread?

Trichomoniasis is primarily spread through sexual contact, which includes vaginal, penile, or vulvar contact.

3. What are the symptoms and indicators of trichomoniasis?

 Itching, burning, abnormal discharge, and discomfort during urination are all possible symptoms. A significant number of cases, however, are asymptomatic.

4. How is trichomoniasis diagnosed?

Clinical evaluation, laboratory tests (such as wet mount microscopy or nucleic acid amplification tests), and physical examination are all part of the diagnosis process.

5. Can trichomoniasis be asymptomatic?

 Yes, a significant number of people with trichomoniasis might not experience any symptoms.

6. How is trichomoniasis treated?

Trichomoniasis is treated with prescription medications, most notably metronidazole or tinidazole, which are administered orally or intravaginally.

7. Can trichomoniasis be cured?

Yes, trichomoniasis can be cured with proper and timely treatment. Both sexual partners should be treated at the same time.

8. What happens if trichomoniasis is not treated?

Untreated trichomoniasis can result in complications such as an increased risk of other STIs, pregnancy complications, pelvic inflammatory disease (PID), and transmission to sexual partners.

9. Can trichomoniasis be transmitted in non-sexual ways?

No, trichomoniasis is primarily a sexually transmitted infection that is not spread by casual contact or shared items.

10. How soon after trichomoniasis exposure do symptoms appear?

Symptoms may appear 5 to 28 days after exposure, but the incubation period can vary.

11. Can trichomoniasis affect men?

Yes, trichomoniasis can affect men and cause urethritis, with symptoms such as urination discomfort and discharge.

12. Can I contract trichomoniasis from a toilet seat or a swimming pool?

No, trichomoniasis is not spread through shared items such as toilet seats or swimming pools. It is primarily transmitted through sexual contact.

13. Can trichomoniasis be passed on during oral sex?

Trichomonasis can be transmitted during oral sex if infected genital or oral tissues are in contact.

14. Does trichomoniasis affect fertility?

Untreated trichomoniasis and its complications, such as pelvic inflammatory disease (PID), can have an impact on fertility in both men and women.

15. Can condoms prevent trichomoniasis?

Although consistent and correct condom use can reduce the risk of trichomoniasis, it does not provide complete protection.

16. Can I get trichomoniasis more than once?

Yes, individuals can get trichomoniasis more than once especially if both partners are not treated concurrently or if high-risk behaviors persist.

17. Is trichomoniasis transmitted during menstruation?

While the risk is higher during menstruation, trichomoniasis is mostly spread through sexual contact.

18. Does trichomoniasis have a vaccine?

There is currently no vaccine available for trichomoniasis. Safe sexual practices and timely treatment are essential for prevention.

19. Can trichomoniasis be detected using a blood test?

No, trichomoniasis is diagnosed through clinical examination and laboratory tests like wet mount microscopy or nucleic acid amplification.

20. Can pregnant women be treated for trichomoniasis?

Yes, pregnant women can be treated for trichomoniasis, and treatment plans may be adjusted based on individual circumstances and trimesters.

MYTHS AND FACTS ABOUT TRICHOMONIASIS

Trichomoniasis is an infection caused by the protozoan parasite Trichomonas vaginalis that is spread through sexual contact. Unfortunately, trichomoniasis misinformation and myths can contribute to stigma and misunderstandings

Let's bust some myths and provide accurate information:

Myth 1: Trichomoniasis is only found in women.

Fact: Both men and women can get trichomoniasis. While women may experience symptoms such as itching, burning, and discharge, men can develop urethritis and experience symptoms such as urination discomfort and discharge.

Myth 2: You can only get trichomoniasis if you're promiscuous.

Fact: Trichomoniasis is a sexually transmitted infection that can affect anyone who engages in sexual activity. It is not limited to people who have multiple sexual partners.

Myth 3: Trichomoniasis is always symptomatic.

Fact: A significant number of trichomoniasis cases are asymptomatic, which means that people may not notice any symptoms. Asymptomatic infections must be detected through regular screenings.

Myth 4: Trichomoniasis can be spread through shared items such as toilet seats.

Fact: Trichomoniasis is transmitted primarily through sexual contact, rather than through casual contact or shared items such as toilet seats, towels, or swimming pools.

Myth 5: If you use condoms, you can't get trichomoniasis.

Fact: While consistent and correct condom use can reduce the risk of trichomoniasis, it does not provide complete protection. The infection can spread through genital areas that are not covered by condoms.

Myth 6: Trichomoniasis only affects children.

Fact: Trichomoniasis can affect people of all ages who engage in sexual activity. It is not restricted to any particular age group.

Myth 7: Trichomoniasis is synonymous with yeast infection.

Fact: A parasite causes trichomoniasis, while a fungus causes yeast infections. While both can cause vaginal symptoms, they are treated differently.

Myth 8: Trichomoniasis causes infertility.

Fact: Trichomoniasis does not cause infertility. While untreated trichomoniasis can cause complications such as pelvic inflammatory disease (PID), which can have an impact on fertility, prompt treatment can help prevent these complications.

Myth 9: If you're in a monogamous relationship, you can't get trichomoniasis.

Fact: If one partner becomes infected, trichomoniasis can still occur in monogamous relationships. Maintaining sexual health requires regular screenings and open communication.

Myth 10: Trichomoniasis is a minor infection.

Fact: Trichomoniasis, if left untreated, can cause pelvic inflammatory disease (PID), increased susceptibility to other STIs, and pregnancy complications. It is critical to receive treatment as soon as possible.

Myth 11: Herbal remedies can cure trichomoniasis.

Fact: There is no scientific evidence that herbal remedies can cure trichomoniasis. The recommended treatment is prescription medications.

Myth 12: You can't get trichomoniasis if you don't have symptoms.

Fact: Asymptomatic people can still carry and spread trichomoniasis. Regular screenings are required, especially for those who are at higher risk.

It is important to dispel these myths in order to promote accurate information about trichomoniasis, reduce stigma, and promote proactive measures such as regular screenings and safe sexual practices.

Education and open communication are critical in dispelling myths and empowering people to make informed decisions about their sexual health.

CONCLUSION

As the comprehensive exploration of trichomoniasis comes to a close, it becomes clear that understanding this sexually transmitted infection (STI) is critical not only for individuals directly affected, but also for broader public health initiatives. This book's journey through its pages has revealed the many facets of trichomoniasis, from its transmission, symptoms, and diagnosis to the complexities of treatment, partner involvement, and prevention strategies.

Trichomoniasis, caused by the protozoan parasite Trichomonas vaginalis, needs to be addressed because of its prevalence and potential health consequences.

The myth-busting journey dispelled myths about the infection, emphasizing that trichomoniasis does not affect only certain age groups, genders, or relationship dynamics.

Unraveling Trichomoniasis clarified that anyone who engages in sexual activity is vulnerable, and education is critical in eradicating stigma and cultivating a more informed society.

The exploration of the complications and risks associated with untreated trichomoniasis highlighted the importance of prompt intervention. The consequences of ignoring trichomoniasis extend beyond immediate discomfort, ranging from an increased risk of other STIs to potential pregnancy complications. To mitigate these risks and promote long-term well-being, the book emphasized the importance of comprehensive healthcare, partner treatment, and ongoing support.

As we progressed through the chapters, the intricate details of trichomoniasis diagnosis and treatment became clear. Laboratory tests, prescription medications such as metronidazole and tinidazole, as well as dosages and administration instructions, all became integral parts of the story. This knowledge enables people to actively participate in their healthcare journey and encourages healthcare providers to use tailored approaches based on individual needs and circumstances.

Partner treatment has emerged as a cornerstone in trichomoniasis management, emphasizing the interconnectedness of sexual health within relationships. The importance of open communication, empathy, and practical guidance in assisting individuals and their partners through the treatment process was emphasized in the chapters. Also, prevention strategies revealed avenues for reducing trichomoniasis incidence through education, safe sexual practices, routine screenings, and community outreach.

In essence, "Unraveling Trichomoniasis" is a guide to fostering a culture of sexual health awareness, destigmatizing STIs, and promoting preventative measures. It is a valuable resource for individuals seeking clarity, healthcare providers wishing to provide informed care, and communities wishing to live in a healthier environment. Finally, the pages of this book unfold a story that goes beyond the complexities of a single infection, advocating for a comprehensive approach to sexual health and well-being.